MORE JOURNEYS
DOWN THE PATH

More Journeys Down The Path

Edward Neu, MD

Library of Congress Control Number:		2013923732
ISBN:	Hardcover	978-1-4931-5911-6
	Softcover	978-1-4931-5910-9
	Ebook	978-1-4931-5912-3

This book was printed in the United States of America.

Rev. date: 01/02/2014

To order additional copies of this book, contact:
Xlibris LLC
1-888-795-4274
www.Xlibris.com
Orders@Xlibris.com
142340

CONTENTS

Prologue 7

Chapter One: A Happy Addition...9
Chapter Two: A New Idea 12
Chapter Three: A Full Existence..15
Chapter Four: The Aftermath 19
Chapter Five: The Next Couple of Weeks 23
Chapter Six: The Second Debate: Dreams...................................27
Chapter Seven: A Visit with the Doctor 31
Chapter Eight: A Dream...34
Chapter Nine: The Third Meeting: Out-of-Body Experiences 38
Chapter Ten: An OBE 41
Chapter Eleven: A Working Weekend...44
Chapter Twelve: Another OBE Experience 47
Chapter Thirteen: A View of Time...50
Chapter Fourteen: Another Visitation 53
Chapter Fifteen: Encephalopathy 56
Chapter Sixteen: Another Bleeding Episode.................................59

Epilogue: A Conversation 63

Prologue

He was ready. Everything was in place. The spirit entities that he interacted with regularly were in place where they needed to be as his parents. His relationships with them had been in other positions in their episodes together, sometimes altering relationships. Son could be mother or father, as could the others make switches.

This time he was going to be their son, and all three, along with supporting characters, were ready for Sean to enter the physical world. He started his journey toward birth and let out a bloodcurdling cry as he turned his awareness to the physical world with its bright lights and noises.

CHAPTER ONE

A Happy Addition

Mary was sitting up between contractions. She had been at it for about eight hours, and they were happening every three to four minutes. The doctor had said she was making progress, but to her, she would like to have been done with this several hours ago. Another contraction hit, and she did her best to breathe correctly. Like many others, she was quietly thinking about never wanting to go through this ever again. But she knew if they had the opportunity and Joe felt like having more children, she would do it again. Another contraction started, and she worked her way through it.

Joe was constantly at her side, encouraging her and rubbing wherever it helped. He was totally grateful to her for wanting to have his child. He just hoped that he could keep up with the baby and, later on, his teenager. He promised himself that he would do his best for the child and raise someone with good intentions and morals.

Mary began feeling the urge to push with her contractions, but when she was checked, she was told to hold off on any pushing but that she was almost ready for that stage. After another half an hour, she was told to start pushing with her contractions, and the character of her contractions changed. Soon the baby's head was presenting, and she pushed a little longer before the shoulder presented. With one last contraction, the baby was delivered in good condition, and they had a new baby boy in their family.

The baby was healthy, and the rest of the delivery went well. Mary felt much better, with tears in her eyes. They gave her the baby to hold for a few minutes, and she was overwhelmed and in tears.

The baby was placed in an incubator to keep warm, and Mary was carted off to her hospital room from the delivery room where she had been for the past half hour. The day was young, it being early in the morning, and Mary was exhausted. She was allowed a nap before seeing the baby again to try to start feeding him.

Joe was on the phone with Mary's parents to tell them the happy news. He also called a colleague who was responsible for getting the news out to Joe's friends.

By the next couple of visits, a successful routine of feeding the baby had been established. Mary was ready for discharge from the hospital, and they went home where the feeding routine was continued while Joe tried to keep Mary comfortable and fed her.

Joe thanked Mary often and was elated to be at home with them because he had his seasoned present hematology fellow, John, cover the patient load in the hospital for him and keep him informed about any new issues at the hospital. Everything seemed to go smoothly with that arrangement. John was in his second and last year of hematology fellowship and was trusted by Joe to handle any clinical issues or at least know when to lean on Joe for some answers when he needed some help. This kept things on Joe's service under control, leaving Joe the chance to take a couple of days off to spend with Mary and the baby. They decided to name the boy Sean to reflect some of Mary's Irish ancestry. All was well with the world, and Joe was elated to have his new child home and healthy. He did the best he could to keep Mary happy, fed, and comfortable.

When Joe did get back to work, he was greeted with cheers when he first saw his fellow and some of the medical residents with whom he also worked. They were happy for him, knowing his medical condition of chronic sarcoidosis and how that affected him.

The sarcoidosis mainly affected his stamina these days, limiting the hours he could spend teaching his fellow and the medical residents. Joe had a contract with the residency program to do teaching rounds with the residents that he worked with in a rotating manner. Then he had his fellow to teach, though John was more of a help than a time drain. He usually took the consults throughout the hospital and then discussed them with Joe, so he was happy to have John around for the past several months as a second-year hematology fellow.

Joe also was in pain due to a peripheral neuropathy felt mostly in his legs when he stood long or tried to walk very far, so he conserved his energy when it came to walking. Joe just seemed to fatigue easily, so he had to watch his pace and take breaks when he needed to. He was considered an asset to the teaching program though, so he was accepted for what he could bring to the teaching of the residency program. He also was an asset to the hospital just because he was a good physician when it came to patient care.

At times when he was at the hospital, he would think about Mary and the new baby at home, and that seemed to keep his work easier to perform because those thoughts of his family seemed to give him more energy. Mary planned to return to her nursing job after the baby was a couple of months old. She had been able to enlist her mom to help with watching and caring for the baby while she worked at the hospital part-time or a couple days a week. Her mom lived nearby and was elated to be involved in helping to care for the child when both Joe and Mary worked or even wanted an early evening out together.

Once the routine was established, it felt to Mary like she had been doing this for a long time even though it had been going on for just a few weeks, and Mary was feeling better reestablishing her relationship with her coworkers. She was happy to be back to work, interacting with adults again after spending 95 percent of her time without adult stimulation other than Joe and her mother. It felt good to talk to some of her friends at work to help reduce the feeling of isolation.

She found herself loving Joe even more now that they had a physical symbol of their love for each other in Sean's presence. To her, Joe seemed happier with the baby's existence as well. Joe was sure to tell Mary often that he loved her because he felt much closer to her now that they had Sean with them as part of the family.

Chapter Two

A New Idea

Joe and his fellow, John, stopped for some lunch after a couple of hours rounding. Tom, a second-year medical resident, and Dave, his intern, joined them at the lunch table. Joe and John had seen them earlier to evaluate an anemic person on Tom's service.

Joe had been thinking about bringing back the talks like he had had a few years earlier during his residency, where the participants would pick a medical or metaphysical topic to discuss in debate format and open it to anyone wanting to join the group. He stated to the others, "I have been thinking about bringing back the talks we had once before where we debate the important things in life and death. I think we should allow anyone into the group who wants to join us. We could hold them here at the hospital so the largest group could attend and join in the discussions. If we have them, we may get some attending doctors to attend, as many of them are off and probably playing golf, but maybe they would check us out. I could think about a couple of topics relating to my baby Sean, but there are other topics as well."

John replied, "I wasn't there for the first discussions, but I heard about them, and I think it would be a good idea. We could schedule them toward the end of the day shift so that the most people would get a chance to join us if they wanted to."

The others agreed too, and they decided to talk to the program director to see if they could institute the idea. Joe said he would get back to them after he discussed it with Dr. Jones, the medical residency program director.

When they finished lunch, Joe put in a call to Dr. Jones and had him paged so Joe could discuss the idea with him. No sooner had Joe reached the ninth floor than Dr. Jones was on the phone answering him. Joe discussed his idea, and Dr. Jones agreed to let Joe go ahead and develop it, and he offered Joe the use of the small auditorium if he wanted it, depending on the interest in the project.

Once Joe got off the phone, he relayed the news to Tom and Dave about Dr. Jones's support for the discussions. Joe then suggested they try to enlist other medical and surgical residents who might have an interest in the talks and that they try to arrange a time midafternoon on a Friday in two weeks to have their first meeting and that they try life before birth or after death as a topic. "My son Sean has been with us for approximately three months now, and before he came here, was there something of him, a soul, existing among us, waiting for an entry to our physical world or realm? Where does one end up after they leave this existence and die?

"I can tell you that when I had my heart stopped on the operating table, I did not bring back any memory of my time 'dead,' before I was revived, after I returned to the living, though instances have been reported in the literature of people remembering being out of their body during surgical procedures gone wrong with heart stoppage and then being revived."

John, Joe's fellow, said, "I'll take the existence of a nonphysical life, if Tom here will take the nonexistence of a nonphysical life side." As Joe's fellow, John always felt the need to do his best to impress Joe because his successful graduation and status as a member of a completed fellowship program completely depended on Joe's recommendation for membership into the community of hematology fellows. Tom agreed with the proposal, and they set a tentative date to meet on Friday three weeks away.

They got back to work. Joe and John went off to see a consultation regarding excessive bruising in a patient on the ninth floor, and Tom, with his intern, went back to their floor to check a new admission to their service—a person suffering sepsis who was currently at the emergency room.

Joe had a chance to check on Mary to see how her day was going before they looked at their consultation. "It's been steady but workable today," she stated. "I'm under control."

John went in to see the patient, a thirty-five-year-old woman with extensive bruising over her arm, legs, and abdomen. There was also a question of some spleen enlargement upon examination. Joe had gone over the chart labs while John had been busy seeing the patient. Joe trusted John's exam skills but took a few minutes to introduce himself to the patient and to do a quick physical exam on her before he got together with John to discuss their findings.

John mentioned the bruising and enlarged spleen, and Joe concurred, then relayed the lab abnormalities. The patient had a mild megaloblastic anemia with somewhat low platelets and a prolonged blood clotting tests and a mildly abnormal kidney function test. Joe asked John what he thought. John replied, "It fits thrombotic thrombocytopenic purpura, or TTP. But could it be something else?"

Joe responded, "When it quacks like a duck, it's a duck. But why does she have it? Did you notice the slight confusion that she has? She couldn't name the hospital she was in or tell me the date, so that also fits in with the TTP."

John replied, "There could be an underlying infection setting off the TTP process, and treatment would be antibiotics and supportive fluids to try to avoid the next step in the disease process or septic shock, which could develop without treatment. I would pan-culture her and start broad-spectrum antibiotics."

Joe responded, "I agree, and we should move quickly. I'll write some orders for the nurse and give the consulting service a call."

Once that had been taken care of, Joe and John had some free time, so they stopped at the library, Joe to check out the latest hematology journals and John to research his topic for the discussion coming up soon.

Joe had placed an information and sign-up sheet for the debate on life between physical existences and found that several people signed up to take part or at least to watch the discussion, so he hoped everything would go smoothly once they got started with what he considered to be a series of debates. He wanted the series to be a success, especially because it would start at the onset of the new resident year, July 1. Sean had been born in March, which made him a Pisces, and he was now going on his fourth month of life. What little Joe knew of astrology, Pisces individuals were supposed to be "old souls" or came from a place or time where old souls were conceived.

Joe's workday was coming to an end and not too soon for him. He was a little tired out from their work that day, and he went up to see how Mary was doing. She had given her report to the evening nurse and was just finishing up, so they left together to go home. They ate some spaghetti with some sauce Joe had put together the day before, anticipating wanting a simple dinner after a nearly full day of work.

When they were done, Mary cleared the table and then met Joe on the couch to sit together for some television. After the news, they went to the bedroom after settling Sean hopefully for the night and snuggling in together under the sheet. They hugged and kissed for a little while before drifting off to a sound sleep.

CHAPTER THREE

A Full Existence

Sean was changing daily, interacting with them in expanding ways. It was now early in July, and they were constantly catching themselves spoiling the boy. He was sleeping well, which helped their sleep schedule. On nice days, they would take him for a ride in the stroller, and he often fell asleep. The quietness and pleasantness of those periods of sleep were coveted by each of them.

One day during one of their trips around the block, Joe told Mary about starting the debates like they had done before during their residency years. Joe mentioned that he wanted to give it a try.

It came to the day before their first session, centered on the question of where Sean was before he was born, or what occurs before birth and what occurs at death and after death. Joe reminded Mary about it and said he hoped she could stop by to see part of it. "John is going to take the 'something happens and exists' side of the argument, and Tom is going to take the 'there is nothingness until fertilization' side. I am off tomorrow except for phone calls, so I can go over there just before or a little earlier if I want to check on anyone there for the meeting."

Mary responded, "Of course, I'll be there to see it. I was promised by my supervisor that I can come down for a while. I just hope that this doesn't get to be too much for you."

Joe replied, "We are just going to do it every three weeks, so I don't think it will be too taxing. The worst thing would be that I start a little later on Thursday to stay rested."

Mary retorted, "Well, break a leg."

Joe answered, "Thanks a lot."

They gave each other a kiss and hugged for a while. Sean was sleeping well in the next room. When Joe rolled onto his back, Mary snuggled next to him with her head on his chest. He began going over how he planned to open up the class or meeting and the moderating of it. Once he was satisfied, he drifted off to sleep.

The next morning, Joe arose with Mary because he decided he wanted to use the library at the hospital for a while. He was going to drive her to work anyway. When it was time, they hopped in the car and drove to the hospital. They said good-bye in the parking lot because Joe was going to use a different door than Mary. So they went their separate ways until their agreed-upon lunch together. Joe ended up using the library until it was time for his class.

He walked to the auditorium and set some notes on the podium. The class had about fifteen people signed up. He figured that would be fine while they tried the first discussion or two, and he expected word of mouth to bring new people each session.

A few minutes after the starting time, they were short just a couple of medicine residents who ended up showing up a little late. So he started the class by leaving the podium and sitting in a chair facing the others. He discussed his goals for and the format of the class. "We are modeling these discussions much after the meetings we started during my last year of residency several years ago. We enjoyed our time with the talks and have attempted to use the same rules that we used then. The participant 'volunteers' but is often given the side of the argument most likely against the person's personal views.

"We continue until both sides agree to quit or a time is selected to finish the discussion. Everyone is involved. Questions from the audience are encouraged, and with that, I introduce Doctors John and Tom. John is pro, and Tom is con today. I'll give the floor to John to start his argument of the question."

John rose and, while standing, began, "Where is an entity or spirit before birth? It is hearsay from self-proclaimed psychics that the soul picks the family he or she goes to because of a cycle between entities that seem to reappear together as a group. The relationships may be changed each time, but they seem to stay together. Likewise, after physical death, the entities are said to congregate again to compare notes, so to speak. This is discussed by several different psychics or mediums. It seems to coincide with previous stories each time you pick up a different psychic who has a book for you to read. So the nonphysical portion of our life cycle appears to be active and filled with information to assimilate.

"There are, of course, books reporting out-of-body experiences, either spontaneous or induced, which bring back stories, some verifiable, about objects seen on the other side of the world. This suggests extra unknown communication or insights available to the people who have control of it and can report the findings back to the physical body or brain.

"So I am proposing that a lot occurs during our inattention to the physical life, and by highlighting looking inward, the information can be available to anyone who learns how to retrieve and process it.

"At this time I will give the floor to Tom." John sat down as Tom rose and pulled his chair forward to sit back down on it. His attempt was to look different from John, more relaxed.

"Well, I believe that it is like this. Two gametes merge and create a unique DNA pattern, which then starts dividing, producing more cells, and life begins. A child forms due to instructions in the DNA pattern, and it is born after thirty-nine or forty weeks ideally, and he grows into a Sean based on his DNA instructions.

"This individual is then molded by his experiences and surroundings. Much of what he is, is motivated by reaction to physical elements in his life and situations that he encounters.

"I yield the chair back to John." With that, Tom rose, pulled his chair back, and sat back down.

John stood and began, "There must be more to life than mere chemical reactions in a physical organism, though I can see someone mistakenly believe that that is what we are, a collection of chemical reactions which holds us together. Those who profess that they can talk to the dead are getting information from somewhere, from something that knows about the dead person. Who better to give the information than the dead person? In order for that to take place, the medium must contact someone or something who knows things about the dead person. There must be something, like a spirit entity, holding the dead person's own personal experiences, and this we can refer to as the soul or spirit body. I don't know how else the medium can come up with the information that he does about the dead person.

"Have you ever been contacted by someone you love in a dream? These experiences are common and often verifiable. It happens that something is said or referred to during these readings that someone in the family can relate directly to the dead person.

"There must be an entity that relates to the dead person's life, as it is known by those who proceed along in life, after the representative appearing to be the dead person's spirit lives on in a spirit world or 'heaven' as it is believed to be by some people.

"I believe that the entity or soul continues on after death and reevaluates his or her previous life in preparation for more learning the next time it manifests physically. It is involved in the selection process of what it will learn by experience in the next life. It also reviews what it learned in the life just experienced."

John took a break by stating, "I will yield the chair back to Tom unless there are any questions at this time."

A hand went up, and Dr. Jones was recognized. "What is involved in the selection process for the next physical experience?"

John replied, "The entity or soul meets with helper souls who review his past life with him and discuss what he wants to learn the next time. He is then aided in selecting a role which will allow him a chance to learn a life lesson during his next visit here. That generally explains what happened with us, as well as with Sean just before he came to live with Joe and Mary."

With that he sat, and Tom rose, this time staying on his feet. He began his retort. "We have a lot to assimilate here, but it is just as possible that these nonphysical actions and thoughts could be just a vivid imagination. There is no reason to need to create all of these nonphysical machinations. It is much easier to just accept that when two gametes meet, a life is started, and it continues until it ceases to exist."

Tom ended with that, and the discussion was opened for questions. Once they were covered, the class adjourned for the day, and everyone filed out of the room. Joe received a few comments from some of those present as they left. They were mostly positive and asking for the next topic. Joe stated that the next meeting would be in three weeks, and the topic would be posted in the doctors' lounge and cafeteria once it was chosen. After the room cleared, he looked for Mary and found her. They walked to the car and headed home. They decided to pick up some fast food on the way home.

Mary told Joe that she had seen the whole meeting and enjoyed it, but she asked Joe how he was feeling.

Joe replied, "I felt more alive doing that. I really enjoyed it, and I think it went well."

They arrived at home and carried their food in to devour it in front of the television news. Mary gave Joe a kiss and said she was happy that Joe had gone ahead with his debate project as he seemed to really enjoy it.

They went to bed a little early because Joe was tired, but they took some time to cuddle before drifting off to sleep for the night.

CHAPTER FOUR

The Aftermath

The next morning, Mary got up and showered before checking on Joe. He was just getting up as she saw him. "I think I am going to go in around noon today. I feel a little more tired today than I expected to be. Can you get yourself to work this morning? I'll be okay, but I'm going to take it easy this morning. We don't have too much going on today."

Mary replied, "Are you sure you're okay? Maybe yesterday was too much."

Joe answered, "What I can do is—since John was in the middle of the debate yesterday, he knows how the class works—I could have him take over as moderator, and I can take a minimal role in the meeting with less stress."

Mary agreed, "That sounds like a good idea."

Joe's chronic aches and pains were a bit worse today, a sign that he might have done too much yesterday. He got up and hopped into the shower before saying good-bye to Mary. He told her he would stop by the ninth floor to see her when he got to the hospital.

Mary replied, "Okay." She gave him a kiss and left for work.

Joe took his time getting something to eat and then checked out the computer to see what was going on in the world and to check his mail, which he hadn't done for a couple of days. He called John to see if anything new was going on. John mentioned a new consult regarding anemia but said that he would take care of it before Joe got there. John was a good asset to have, and they communicated well with each other. Joe was sure that John would make a good physician and hematologist when he finished his training.

By noon he was ready to go to the hospital and get some hands-on work done. As promised, when he got there, he tracked down Mary to say hi to her. Then he met with John, who told him that he had already done a bone marrow biopsy on the new anemic consult that they had. By tomorrow they would get some preliminary results. They discussed the case a little further, and Joe told John that he was on the right track.

In some ways, Joe's lack of energy left him hoping that this didn't happen too regularly as he felt useless to do anything himself. John had seen their patients already, and they discussed how everyone was doing. The woman with the bruising was improving, but she had grown some bacteria in her blood and urinary bladder, so her ultimate cause in the bruising was TTP due to gram-negative sepsis, which was being treated with the IV antibiotics that they had started. Her kidneys were working fine, so they felt that she would do well without further problems.

He limped through the afternoon and was ready to leave work by the time that Mary was finished, so they left her car in the parking lot and went home together in Joe's car. Joe asked Mary if she was up for a Cobb salad with a little chicken in it for dinner. He felt that cutting back on the meat protein for a while might be helpful in regaining his energy. It would help in clearing his mind as well. She agreed that that would be good, so when they got home, he pulled a chicken breast out of the freezer to panfry. He placed some on a couple of plates and took it into the living room where Mary and Sean were still sitting on the couch. Sean had been fed by Mary's mom before they got home, so they all sat together, and Mary and Joe enjoyed their dinner.

The next day was Friday, and Joe had teaching rounds with the resident service that he was supervising, so he went to bed a little early to try to catch up on some sleep and hopefully feel better for the sake of his class. Mary put Sean to bed but stayed up a little longer watching some late-night television as she wasn't quite ready to go to bed yet. She was proud that Joe's new class went well and hoped that he could continue it because he did seem to enjoy it. She did go to bed after an hour or so and found Joe deeply asleep. Mary crawled into bed without disturbing Joe and went to sleep quickly.

In the morning, they arose together and went off to the hospital in Joe's car. Mary went off to the ninth floor, and Joe caught up with John to make rounds together. He was feeling significantly better. After rounds, they stopped down in pathology to see if the bone marrow biopsy was ready to look at. It was, so they had it retrieved for them to view. The slide showed increased fibrosis of the marrow with little red cell production. To them it looked like myelofibrosis, a myelodysplastic syndrome with periods of decreased red blood cell production, like it was happening to their patient. At other times, the marrow would produce too many red blood cells, and it was called polycythemia vera. The treatment in the stage that their patient was in while anemic was blood transfusions, while in the other state it was removing pints of blood or medication. The disease could at times turn into a form of leukemia, so the patient needed to be monitored for all the possibilities. They decided that they wanted the official pathological report before they talked to the patient about it, but they could give her a couple pints of blood to improve his signs and symptoms of fatigue.

Joe had to meet the residents on the seventh floor first thing in the afternoon, so he met with Mary for a quick lunch. She asked him, "How are you feeling?"

He replied, "Pretty good. After teaching rounds, I'll be mostly done for the day, so I think I will be fine."

She said, "Good, but do only what you have to do. Keep things to a minimum, then we can go to bed a little early again tonight."

He agreed, and since they were finished, he asked if she was ready to go. She was, so they stood and walked to the elevators. Joe said good-bye at the seventh floor, and Mary disembarked on the ninth floor to restart her work.

The residents were ready for Joe, so they got started right away. Joe had them go through each of the patients and offered insights along the way. They discussed one of their more difficult patients with Joe, and he gave them his opinion. After about an hour and a half, Joe gave them the bed number of his patient with myelofibrosis and told them to evaluate the patient for teaching rounds the next time on Monday. He wanted them to look up the disease and have one of them present the case to him.

He figured he had about an hour before Mary would finish her work and decided that he didn't really need to do anything else for the day, so he went to the library to read a couple of journals. Just after three thirty, he went up to catch up with Mary and suggested that they just take one car again and they could talk about things on the way home. She said, "We could always talk on the phone on the way home."

He responded, "You're bad. You don't use the phone while you are driving, do you?"

She replied, "Probably once or twice in my life when it was necessary, but I don't do it, not for a few years at least."

He retorted, "Okay, just don't do it anymore, you're a mother."

They got home, and Joe had made some sauce with zucchini for meatless spaghetti, again, to keep the meat protein down. They both greeted Sean when they saw him and got a big smile back. Mary fed Sean while Joe heated up the sauce and boiled some pasta. They both finished at the same time, so they brought a couple of filled plates to the living room, and placing Sean on the floor by them, they started eating their spaghetti. They left the television off as it was early, and they could then talk to each other.

Joe said, "So today was better than yesterday. I guess I have to pace myself and try to get a little extra sleep."

Mary responded, "Hopefully you're right and that is all it is. But if I tell you that I think you're overdoing things, please listen to me. I want you around for a while, you know."

Joe responded, "Okay, I'll listen, thanks."

Mary removed their plates, taking them to the kitchen, and came back to cuddle as Joe turned on the television to watch news and then one of their favorite programs.

After a while, they decided to go to bed and get another good night's sleep. Joe told Mary, "Tomorrow is my usual short day. We just make rounds and deal with any phone calls at home, so I think I am going to make it through the week."

Mary responded, "Good. Come home early and maybe try a little nap, and maybe you'll feel better through the evening."

Joe replied, "Sounds like a plan."

They kissed and hugged for a bit before rolling to the left to sleep together. Sean was sound asleep in his crib.

CHAPTER FIVE

The Next Couple of Weeks

The next morning, they decided to go in separate cars because Joe was going to just do rounds and then come back home. He had some mail to catch up on and figured he would have time to do that. There were also some letters to write, one evaluating John's fellowship experience at the hospital.

He finished rounds without much trouble and then said good-bye to Mary. He drove home and got himself something to eat before getting at his projects. Writing the note about John got Joe to thinking about getting to know John better. He decided to talk to Mary about it.

When she got home, Joe had started on a stir-fry with shrimp for dinner. He had the food ready to cook, so it was nearly done being prepared. It just needed a quick fry and some rice. After he handed Sean to Mary, he and Mary sat down for a bit to discuss their day. Joe mentioned that he thought that they should invite John over for dinner next week to try to get to know him better socially and personally. Mary agreed that that would be a good idea and that it would be good to know him better. "He seems like a really nice man, it would be nice to know what he plans for himself."

Joe decided to ask him tomorrow about next Saturday's dinner at his house, with John's significant other if she would like to come. John said he would ask if that was good for her and would get back to Joe tomorrow. Joe was happy with that. They finished rounds and left the hospital to enjoy the rest of the day.

Joe got home, and they decided to go to the grocery store for a few things. Joe wanted to try to limit the meat proteins, so they bought more pasta and vegetables. He felt that they could help with his energy and maybe clear his thinking just a little bit. He promised himself that he would make a few good hamburgers and chicken breasts if John came over, and he would select a small chicken breast to eat. He wanted to give the change in diet a try for a while to see if he or Mary could see a difference in his thought processes.

Joe decided to make some panfried chicken for dinner tonight, so he made them when Mary was ready to eat. She fed Sean to make him happy, and then they sat down in the dining room for a change of venue and ate their dinner while Joe talked about his day and conversation with John. He felt that John would probably take them up on their offer.

They spent the evening together on the couch just talking about life and other things as they came to mind. After feeding Sean again, he was put to bed, and they soon followed suit. Joe thought it would be nice to go to bed more awake for a change so they could spend time with each other. They helped each other out of their clothes and climbed into bed together. They proceeded to make love like they used to when they were younger. Mary was impressed, and Joe just said it must be all the good healthy living that she was forcing on him.

They held each other until they fell asleep. Joe had a good night's sleep and felt good when he got up in the morning to do patient rounds and then coming back home after a couple of hours.

The rest of the day was free for relaxing or a leisurely read of the Sunday newspaper. Mary allowed Joe the time to relax because he had made it through a rough week. He spent some time reading the paper to Sean, who was sitting on his lap. Sean seemed just to enjoy hearing him speaking and would giggle at times at some of Joe's exaggerated inflections.

They didn't do anything taxing that day, and late in the afternoon, Joe made pizza with mushrooms and green peppers for dinner. When the pizza was finished, they sat down to have some while watching television. It was satisfying enough by itself, and they felt pleasantly full when they were finished. When it got to be late enough, Sean was put to bed on a full stomach, and they went off to the bedroom for a quiet night's sleep. Joe fell asleep quickly after cuddling and kissing Mary for a little while. Snuggling with her just made him feel good and relaxed him well so that he drifted off to sleep easily with Mary in his arms. Mary dropped off to sleep shortly after Joe.

The next morning seemed to come too quickly for Joe, but they arose and showered together before getting a bite to eat. Then they were off to work together. Joe dropped Mary off with a kiss before parking the car and entering the hospital to find John. He had started rounds on the seventh floor and was about to go to the ninth floor when Joe found him. They went to nine together and finished their rounds there. Everything seemed to go smoothly. The afternoon was filled with teaching rounds, and he had one of the residents present the case of myelofibrosis, which they then discussed at length. Once Joe finished his teaching rounds, he was about done for the day.

It was just a little while before Mary was done, so he told her that he would be in the library when she finished and to come and find him there. She did, and they left to go home for the evening. When they got home, Sean was happy to see them, and he showed it by laughing and smiling whenever he saw them move by or pick him up for a while. Mary felt like fixing dinner, and Joe willingly let her while he spent some time with Sean. They discussed their day. Joe was able to tell Mary that John and his friend Julia would come to dinner on Saturday, and they could have something like the pizza again to feed them. Maybe he could add some pepperonis to one side of it for more choices. Mary was happy to hear that they were coming over. Joe could then ask John about moderating the debate class as well.

The week went smoothly, and Joe had picked another topic for the debate class. He posted it, stating that they were going to talk about the nature and purpose of dreaming. People were to sign up if they were coming. It didn't take long for him to have at least twenty signatures. He selected a couple of residents to be the debaters, and his next class was all set in about two weeks for a session. The residents Bob and Sandy, from other services, had been volunteered to be the arguers for the meeting.

Saturday evening came around, and John arrived at their house with his friend Julia. Though Joe didn't drink, it was offered to John and his friend. Out of deference to Joe, they both declined. Joe told them that he had a pizza ready to go into the oven for dinner, which sounded good to John. While it was cooking, Joe took the opportunity to talk to John about his plans for the future. John replied that he really just wished to try private practice but would probably enjoy a teaching position part-time in a university setting. He hoped to stay in the area that they lived in now. He really didn't want to have to move as they were pretty settled where they were. Joe said, "You never know." There could be a position opening soon where he was because he wasn't sure how much longer he was going to be able to work and teach with his condition.

John said they would talk more about that, but he felt that Joe was still doing pretty well.

Joe replied, "I have my good days and bad days."

John said that Janet wanted to stay in the area too because all her family lives in the area. They would at least get some help from her family, much like Joe and Mary were getting from her mother. That was always a plus with having family around.

When their discussion was over, Joe felt that John might be the right person to groom to take his position when he couldn't work anymore. He didn't see that he was going to work all that much longer as even the light days seemed to wear him out at times.

Mary got to know Janet a little. She had come from a large family and hoped for the same with her family when she started one. She presently worked as a legal secretary and could pick her work hours when she got around to having children. So they were pretty well situated with their two incomes.

When the pizza was ready, they stopped talking and started on the pizza, devouring it almost completely. When dinner and discussion were over, John and Janet said good night and left to drive home to their so-far-empty apartment.

Later on, Joe remembered this night as a turning point in John's young career. He began relying more on John and giving him more responsibility. He began discussing his illness with John as well and began to consider him a doctor that he could go to for help in the future if he needed it. In that way, their relationship changed a little.

Chapter Six

The Second Debate: Dreams

The day for the second debate arrived, and people began filling the auditorium seats a little more compared to the first debate. So word of mouth must be catching on, Joe thought. When it came time to start, John appeared to introduce the debaters and the topic.

He started, "Welcome, everybody. Today we have Bob and Sandy, who are going to debate the nature of dreams and what they are for. Our debate leaders today are Sandy, who is in favor of dreams being significant, and Bob, who is going to argue that dreams are of no value other than as an entertaining diversion. I yield the floor to Bob to start today."

John sat down, and Bob rose from his chair on the stage to begin. "Dreams are entertaining, but as usual rehashes of the previous day, they tend to be redundant or boring. Don't you usually find yourself walking around familiar surroundings or running or swimming for fun? Some people feel that dreams are wish fulfillment. You could be driving that car that you saw the day before and thought about owning. In the dream, you do. There are no hidden messages or unusual activities in dreams, except for a little flying at times. They are mainly just entertainment based on everyday input added to your memory the day before. I will yield the floor to Sandy here and let her respond to these insights."

He sat down, and Sandy stood for her opening remarks. "Dreams play an important role in assimilating the previous day's activities and encounters. More insight after a dream is common due to the sorting-out processes in dreaming. Answers to difficult problems being worked on before the dream are often resolved while dreaming. This involves higher brain function while in the dream. Symbols appear often in dreams, like the car mentioned by Bob, which can be a symbol for protection or a symbol for the human body, which houses the soul while we live our physical existence.

"Clairvoyant dreams are referenced in the literature where it is suggested that the future manifests in the dream before it happens. A debate such as this one here can be dreamed about, which helps to organize the situation when it comes to pass in the future of the dream, like dreaming last night of today's debate. With this scenario, one can see dreaming the lottery numbers for the next day's lottery. It's a shame that we don't have more control over dreaming what we want to as we would probably have more lottery winners coming up for prize payouts. There is symbolism in dreams, like dreaming of a key may mean unlocking a mystery, or the car, as mentioned above, could stand for our physical self, and a nonworking or dented part could mean a defect, like engine trouble could mean trouble with one's heart. So interpreted correctly, the dream can give personal insight into our health information, which our subconscious mind has access to and often is the source of our dream subject.

"I will yield the floor back to Bob for comment," said Sandy while sitting back down.

Bob stood and began, "I think that Sandy is giving too much meaning to our dreams. Some consider them to be simple subconscious pleas of wish fulfillment. In the dream, we may get what we have been wanting in our awakened state. They are an escape, flights of fancy where we can play roles different from our daily life. That is the simple truth, they are not messages of the soul, which hasn't been debated here yet as to the very existence of it. They are just entertainment for the idle brain designed by the idle brain during sleep. There isn't much else to say about dreams. I will yield back to Sandy." He sat down, and Sandy stood again.

Once on her feet, Sandy started, "Dreams have been called the window to the soul. Who's to say our subconscious is not in touch with our soul, and these dreams may be messages from our soul about deeper subjects that we don't fully understand when we wake and remember our dreams with some obscure symbols which need interpreting for full understanding. Visitations of dead family members abound in dreams as do visions of the future. What if they are just what they seem to be, visitations or opening of awareness of the future rather than passing them off as wish fulfillment?

"There are methods described that teach one how to control dreams for more effect or understanding. This is used by people who work as problem solvers during their day jobs. Maybe through repetition of sleep and dreaming techniques, they become more adept at it, but the answers to their problems are often worked out in the dream. Insight into the higher levels of consciousness is also available through dreams. The layers of restriction of higher consciousness during the awake period are often loosened during sleep, allowing access to less restricted areas of brain activity. It is in these areas that we have access to the subconscious mind, which we are generally unaware of during waking hours. There is much more going on than we know during dreaming activity. Lucid dreaming occurs when a person gains control of the dream and can control its direction through intention.

"If there are any questions or comments from the audience, we can take them now."

A hand went up from one of the medical residents there, and when acknowledged, George asked, "Are there categorized conventions for certain symbols in dreams?"

Sandy answered, "Yes, Carl Jung spent a lot of time investigating dreaming and supplied several symbols used in dreaming. Like the car used as a symbol for the physical body mentioned earlier, the brain can be seen as a computer or an engineer. The heart can be represented as a pump or as a symbol for true love. Accepted generalized symbols that we have when awake are also used in dreaming, like a dove meaning peace works both in the awake state and in dreams. These symbols are generalized by some and are individual to some people because of the meaning of a special relationship."

John rose and asked, "Are there any other thoughts?"

No one spoke up, so he stated, "I guess for now we are done. Just keep in mind that your dreams may be telling you more than you suspect, so keep an open mind about them. Some people keep a dream diary, which can sometimes help with further understanding of one's dreams on an individual basis. One should give it a try for a while and see what insights may occur. We will adjourn for now. Thanks for coming."

The class broke up and filed through the doors. Joe walked up to John and said, "Thanks for taking this on. I feel that it will do fine with you running it from the moderator position."

John responded with his own, "Thanks for your belief in me."

They walked out together. Joe asked if John would see him as a patient so he could discuss a few things medically with him. John agreed and said they could do it anytime Joe wanted. Joe suggested they do it tomorrow since their workday would be short, and John said it was fine.

The workday ended with the discussion, so Joe found Mary, and they went to the parking lot to pick up the car. Joe suggested that they pick up some fast food for dinner. Joe found and picked up a chicken salad, and Mary selected a chicken sandwich. They then drove home and greeted a smiling Sean, who was clearly happy to see them. Since they had dinner prepared, they were able to spend some time with Sean before they sat down to eat.

They watched the news as they went through their meals, and then they cuddled together with Sean by them for a while until it was time for Sean to eat again and then go off to bed. That accomplished, Mary sat down with Joe again and they cuddled, getting closer while they watched some more television. Joe mentioned to Mary that he was going to see John as a patient tomorrow, partly to discuss his increasing fatigue and painful neuropathy in his legs.

After the news was over, they turned off the television, gave each other a kiss, and moved to the bedroom. Joe was quickly asleep and sleeping soundly through the night.

CHAPTER SEVEN

A Visit with the Doctor

The morning started with them both getting up and taking a shower. They had a bite to eat quickly and then got in the car for their trip to the hospital. Joe caught up with John, and they did rounds together. Then Joe and John went to an outpatient examination room where John could examine Joe.

Joe mentioned his recent fatigue and the constant pain in his legs, especially while on his feet. He seemed a little better after changing his diet recently. Joe had also increased his medicine for encephalopathy, so he felt he was doing okay there. His other main problem was the leg pain, for which he requested something for pain. Because of his condition, there were a lot of things that he couldn't take, so he was given some hydrocodone for when the pain was interfering with his work.

Joe had specialists that he saw for his liver disease and the transplant list that he was on. A lesion seen on his liver was being monitored regularly with CT scans. And his kidneys were watched closely. He just hoped that John could help him with the nonliver parts of his disease. He told John his full history with sarcoidosis and the complications he had had in the past eight or so years since contracting the disease. He then discussed his regular use of pain medication, for which he could use a prescription. Usually, he averaged taking one twice a day unless his legs or back were bothering him more. John wrote him a small prescription for it. He also gave him a note stating his medical use of the drug was given legally to him.

Joe confided with John that he didn't know how much longer he could continue working due to his disability. He said he would give his practice to John when he couldn't work anymore.

John replied, "Thanks, and we will keep you going strong as long as we can. You still have some good years left. Your concentrating ability has been unaffected by the sarcoidosis."

"Well," Joe replied, "when you finish training, you have a job at my clinic and office if you want it."

John said, "Thanks."

Joe checked on Mary. She still had a few hours of work but was about to go down for lunch if he was interested. He said that he would accompany her for that. While at lunch, he told her about his visit with John and how nice he seemed with his bedside manner. He said that John would make a good addition to his office and clinic work.

Mary asked, "How did he do with your symptoms of fatigue?"

Joe replied, "He tried to charm me. He said I still have a few years in me. We'll see."

Mary answered, "You never know what you have left. You are in uncharted waters. No one knows what you have left. I am planning more than a few years."

Joe agreed, resigned. No one could actually know what he had left. His case was unique. "Anyhow, can you think of anything that we need at the grocery store? I was thinking of going there between now and when you get out of work."

"No, not really, we could use some fish to sauté or bake one night," she replied.

Joe went off to the grocery store and was able to stop home to unload before going back to the hospital to pick up Mary. They then went home to relax with Sean before starting a fish dinner. Once the news was over, Mary baked the fish and made some rice and vegetables. Joe took the plates to the kitchen and returned to meet Mary at the couch where they sat together after Mary had picked up Sean and put him between them. The rest of the evening was quiet. They put Sean to bed and went to their room to crawl into bed as well. They gave each other a good-night kiss, and they hugged each other before drifting off to sleep.

They awakened together on Friday and got ready for Joe to drive them to the hospital. Joe's plan was to get there and round on his patients with John before he met with the medical residents for teaching rounds at 10:00 AM. The residents were ready for him when he hit the ninth floor to look for them. They sat down and initially went through their patient list. Then the intern presented the patient that Joe had them see. After that, she gave some pertinent information on myelofibrosis and polycythemia. Joe asked for questions, and after they discussed it for a bit, Joe declared teaching rounds ended. He had the afternoon free, so he spent it in the library. Mary found him there—deeply immersed in an article—when she finished work, so she said hi. He got out of reading the magazine, and they drove home. They spent the evening quietly with Sean and went off to bed after the news.

Saturday, the next day, he just went into the hospital for quick rounds. He didn't see John, but he needed to talk to him in the early afternoon about giving the myelofibrosis patient some more blood, and maybe she could go home tomorrow. "If her hematocrit is over thirty, then send her home," he told John. He had a chance to confirm the time when John and his date would come by for dinner with them.

Dinner started shortly after John and his friend arrived. Joe had prepped the pizza, so he just put it in the oven to cook it. It was Chicago-style deep-dish pizza, so a single pizza ought to be enough, thought Joe. They had a good time chatting while they ate. John was able to tell Mary how much he appreciated Joe's offer to come and work with him in his clinic and his office. He seriously thought about that offer and felt he would probably take Joe up on the offer.

It was getting late, so they decided to end the gathering, and John, with his date, left for the evening. John said he might see Joe tomorrow in the morning while rounding. With that they left, and Mary put Sean to bed for the night. Joe and Mary were ready for bed as well, so they prepared for bed and got under the covers. They chatted a little about the evening and agreed that John felt like a good person and would fit well with Joe in the office and clinic. They kissed and then fell off to sleep.

CHAPTER EIGHT

A Dream

By the time that Joe made rounds the next morning, John had been there already. The patient with the myelofibrosis had a hematocrit of thirty-four, so she had been discharged with an appointment for Joe's clinic in two weeks. She was going to need constant supervision to keep her blood count up, but if caught early enough, she could get a transfusion in the clinic and avoid another hospitalization.

The rest of their patients were dealt with by John already by the time Joe saw them. Joe felt he was probably only an hour or so behind John, but they never did meet, so he settled for a phone call a little later in the morning. Joe thanked John for taking care of most things for their patients, and they left the hospital separately once each had finished their individual rounds.

When Joe got home, he checked on Mary and Sean. Sean was out in his stroller, making himself noticeable by trying a little babbling while he watched Mary doing some weeding in the flower garden that they had near the front of their house. Joe watched them both for a moment before saying hi to let Mary know he was home. He told Mary, "I am going to curl up in my easy chair in the study and take a little nap. I am a little tired."

Mary said, "Okay, we'll be out here so we won't disturb you." She then returned to her weeding.

Joe turned and went to his study where his favorite easy chair was and relaxed into it, closing his eyes. He drifted into a light sleep, and as he was getting drowsier, he began to start thinking about Anna for some reason. As his sleep deepened, Anna came into clearer focus and seemed to be saying something to him. They hugged each other with their greeting. Then Anna showed Joe a picture of him much more encephalopathic, unable to make much sense with his speech, and his thought processes felt more confused.

He awakened with a start, and because it had been so real, he wondered about the information. He was concerned that it meant something, so he decided to call John and discuss it. He hoped that John wouldn't think he was crazy, but it was such a real feeling. Once he had John on the phone, they discussed the patients they saw separately in the morning, but then Joe mentioned his hypnogogic dream and his concerns. John suggested that they follow up with a urine and a couple of blood cultures along with a complete blood count to check for signs of an infection. Joe agreed and told Mary of his dream and his conversation with John.

Mary said she and Sean would drive him to the hospital for the tests, so she cleaned up, and the three of them took a ride to the hospital to get the cultures and blood test and then returned home. When they got there, they checked his temperature, which showed a low-grade fever. Joe took a couple of acetaminophen tablets, which made him feel a little better, but Mary was getting a little concerned because he seemed not to be his usual self.

Later in the afternoon, John called saying that the urine was a little dirty and one of the blood cultures showed a few gram-negative bacteria on a smear. They started a broad-spectrum antibiotic, and John told Joe to stay home from work tomorrow but to stop by and see him so John could check on his mental functioning and he could be sure that Joe wasn't getting any worse.

John was a little concerned when he checked Joe's mental acuity but felt that they had probably caught the infection early. Joe quietly thanked Anna for showing him the infection, if just in a dream.

He talked further about his finding the infection through his dream of Anna. He said, "Who knows if there is anything to it? But I may have been given a warning about the infection by Anna."

Mary agreed that it was unusual but said, "Who knows? If the infection got any worse, you would have ended up in the hospital with sepsis and encephalopathy."

Joe said, "How I discerned the abnormality or I got help from Anna, who knows what happened? But at least I did get some warning very early in the infection, so I will thank Anna."

They stopped to pick up something to eat on the way home because it was dinnertime by the time they got home. Mary fed Sean, and then they ate what they had gotten for themselves. They both got a large salad with a little chicken in it. It was satisfying for both of them, so they went to curl up on the couch to watch television, Joe taking his new antibiotics on schedule.

The next day, Joe decided to stay home and let John do the patient work. He checked in with John later in the afternoon to see if all went well. John mentioned a new consult with anemia. Anemia was one of their most common consults, and frequently it was due to occult bleeding or reduced production of blood for any of a number of reasons. Joe told John that he was feeling a little better and expected to get in to work tomorrow.

John replied, "See how you feel tomorrow. Don't rush getting back, things are under control." Joe tended to get antsy, though, when he had to rest and not work. He expected to go to work just to do something tomorrow. He wasn't going to give in to his disease that easily. With a slight smile on his face, he figured that maybe he was sick with an illness that made him a workaholic. At least there was not a clinical label applied to that defect in his system.

He and Mary went to bed after putting Sean in his crib. After cuddling for a little while, Joe rolled onto his back and thought about what had transpired with his infection. He really felt that he had had contact with Anna and that she was still watching over him. Under his breath, he quietly thanked her for her insight and early intervention, which prevented him from possibly getting very sick.

He closed his eyes after rolling onto his side, facing Mary's back. He gave her a gentle hug, which she didn't feel, sleeping through it, but it was comforting to Joe. He soon joined her in a restful sleep.

When morning came, he arose without difficulty and felt pretty good. The two of them prepared for work, got in the car, and started their trip to the hospital for a day of patient care. When they got to the hospital, Mary went off to the ninth floor, and Joe had John paged so he could catch up with John. On seeing Joe, John took him to a small conference room where they could talk a bit, John assessing Joe's mental sharpness through the conversation. Joe seemed pretty good to John, better than on the phone the day before. They went out and continued the rounds that John had already started.

Joe was feeling tired after rounds, so they sat for a bit, discussing the patients. The bone marrow done on the new consult yesterday would be ready to look at tomorrow. When they had finished their discussion, Joe told John that he was done for the day if John could handle the clinic on his own. John said no problem, so Joe went up to see Mary to tell her he was going home for a while but he would be back to pick her up.

Mary asked, "Are you all right?"

Joe replied, "Yes, just a little tired."

They said their good-byes, and Joe left to go home. He went to lie down on the bed after saying hi to Mary's mother. She had Sean out in the living room with her, so he said hi to Sean as well.

A few hours later, Joe was feeling better, and he drove off to pick up Mary from work. They drove back home for a quiet evening. Mary made something simple for dinner, and they sat down to eat it while watching the news.

Joe went to bed early, and Mary followed suit shortly after. She had stayed up for the nightly news, mainly to check the weather for tomorrow as she was off for the next two days and hoped to get some more work done outside if it wasn't looking like rain. She then crawled into bed without disturbing Joe and slept well.

CHAPTER NINE

The Third Meeting: Out-of-Body Experiences

The subject for the next discussion had been picked. It was on the existence or reliability of out-of-body experiences (OBEs). Bill, a second-year resident, and his intern, Dave, had volunteered to take the two sides of the argument, Bill for the pro side and Dave for the con side. When it came time for the debate, people gathered in the auditorium to hear the discussion, and Bill, Dave, and John took the stage. Joe sat in the back of the room.

When it was time to start, John got up and began, "I am sure that most of us have had the sensation of being somewhere in a room other than where our body is sitting. It lasts just an instant because as soon as we notice it, we are back in our physical body, alert to our surroundings. We are going to discuss that phenomenon today and try to understand it better.

"I will yield the floor to Bill, who is going to speak in favor of the existence of this condition. Dave here is going to take the other side and argue against it being a real experience." With that, John sat down, and Bill rose to his feet to talk. He took out a few papers that had some ideas written on them.

He began, "There are adepts who purport that they can leave the body at will, much as the spirit leaves the body at death. They talk about journeys to great distances or other times at will, usually in an induced trance state sometimes induced by hallucinogenic drugs. The average person though can also have an experience sometimes induced by great stress and sometimes in a meditative state where they can travel to a different place or time. With practice, the experience can be controlled to go to a specific place through intention. There, normal everyday action may be taking place, and they continue to go on without acknowledgement of the traveler because he is invisible to the inhabitants.

"Leaving the body during surgery or in a near-death experience is reported anecdotally. The trips are varied. They can consist of talking to people known to have already passed away or distant traveling to places unseen before but are verifiable as existing in the physical world that we know and live in."

Bill finished by saying, "I will give the floor to Dave for his comments."

Dave rose to his feet and began. "We need to suppose that there is a soul for this process to occur, so let us agree or disagree on that first. If there is no soul, then what is the purpose of our consciousness leaving the body rather than just staying as a physical entity who exists until we die without any ongoing existing nonphysical soul left over? To those nonbelievers, the soul is an unnecessary piece of the puzzle, and we are here for our physical existence, and then we die. All that is of us dies without a separate 'living' soul that accompanies us on our physical journey.

"The soul is an unnecessary creation which is invoked whenever something happens around the death of an individual to explain unexplainable events relating to the death experience. The events can be created by a little wishful thinking on the part of the departed person's friends and relatives to suggest that the departed isn't completely gone but that a part of him still lives on. This extra nonphysical piece of us that lives on is not necessary for our life to be fulfilling."

Dave ended, and as he sat, he said, "I will give the floor back to Bill."

Bill came to his feet again and first asked, "Are there any questions?"

A hand went up in the air, and when recognized, one of the medical residents asked, "Are we going to get to more about out-of-body experiences?"

Bill answered, "I was just about to do that. It is not uncommon for an individual to feel contacted by someone who has just died. These incidents are considered to be visitations. These visits can manifest as dreams. Or during the visitation recipient's awakened state, they may make reference to something especially related to the visitor, like a song or something like that that is easily recognized."

Dave took the floor as Bill motioned to him. He replied, "The visitations have been described as hallucinations brought on by hypoxia related to the dying process or incident causing the situation.

"When the near-death experience occurs to someone, they often experience a pleasant surrounding where they are, whether it is real or imagined. It just makes more sense that it is a hallucination rather than a need to invoke an entire system postdeath that makes a person believe that he has left his body.

"If anyone has any thoughts or questions, they are welcome to stay longer to discuss them with one or both of us."

With that, they adjourned the discussion, and they answered any question before getting up to leave the room. Mary was there and said that she had enjoyed the meeting. She just hadn't been able to go over to sit with him.

He replied, "I think it went pretty well. We got a few thoughts out to think about. If the audience gets that much, then they have gained something."

They were both done with their day at work, so they walked out to the car and picked up something to eat on the way home. After spending some time with Sean, they got him ready for bed and then relaxed together while they watched the nightly news. They soon were ready for bed themselves, so they helped each other out of their clothes. They hugged and kissed for a while and then drifted off to sleep for the night.

Just as Joe was at the edge of sleep, he became very relaxed and began to feel a pleasant vibration go through his body followed by a sense of sliding off the bed onto the floor. The feeling was so real that he opened his eyes to verify where he was. He found himself in his bed, in the same position as when the vibration started. The feeling of movement had been very real to him, however. He moved in the bed and then drifted off to sleep once more.

CHAPTER TEN

An OBE

The next morning came, and they got ready for work and had a bite to eat before getting in the car to go off to work. On the way, Joe related his incident of feeling like he had slid out of bed the night before. "It was so real that I expected to find myself on the floor."

Mary replied, "Maybe you had the beginning of an awake out-of-body experience. If you have that again, let me know. Did you meet anyone?"

Joe answered, "No, but that could be because I didn't go anywhere beyond this room. There could be, and I expect there is, something beyond that room to investigate if I get any more control of the experience."

They drove the rest of the way mostly quietly while they thought about Joe's incident. They both felt that it could have been the beginning of an OBE. Joe just felt that he needed more control over inducing the state and then learning to take more steps toward doing more exploring, going beyond the room to see more.

Once they arrived at the hospital, they went to different directions. Mary went up to the ninth floor, and Joe met John in the pathology department, where the bone marrow biopsy of the patient whom John had biopsied a couple of days earlier was being reviewed by John and a pathologist. After viewing the slides, they visited the patient to tell him that there was an accumulation of abnormal cells in his marrow. They said they would know more later on in the day after some special stains were ready and reviewed.

They suspected lung cancer but wanted a definitive answer before discussing it with the patient. They expected that answer by midafternoon and didn't expect the answer to be good. They went off to make rounds on the rest of their patients. On the ninth floor, Joe was able to catch up with Mary and ask her how her day looked. She reported no surprises, and they agreed to meet for lunch.

Around noon, Joe went to the ninth floor, and then Mary and Joe walked to the cafeteria. After eating some of their lunch, Joe remarked, "I have been thinking about last night, and I can't help reviewing the dream, if that is what it was. It just seemed so real that I wonder if it happened as I remember it."

Mary responded, "It could have been very real. There is no reason to discount it. A view of a nonphysical plane is what you have been talking and thinking about lately. Maybe last night was an affirmation of what has been on your mind lately."

Joe agreed and told Mary he hoped that that dream didn't bother her. She said she was perfectly okay with it, and she hoped he gained more insights into the nature of the experience.

They had finished their lunch, so they got up to go their separate ways. Mary went to the ninth floor, and Joe went to pathology to check on the pathology slides. They did find what looked like a small cell cancer.

Joe had rounds with the residents next, so he went to the ninth floor to track them down. He found Tom and had him track Dave down. Once they were all together, Joe had Tom go through the patients on their service. Joe tried to ask questions that made the residents think. They had gone through the patients, and when they were finished with that, Joe asked the residents if they had any other care questions they wanted to ask. When the questions were all answered, Joe ended the teaching rounds.

Joe went to see the patient and explained the planned treatment and suggested that they get started right away. All risks and benefits were discussed, and Joe ordered treatment after he had the nurse get him a current weight to gauge the dose of chemotherapy drugs to start on.

His work was finished, so he checked with Mary to see how she was doing. She was going to be done soon, so Joe asked her to come find him in the library when she was done. They went home and greeted Sean, who smiled broadly when he saw them. They spent some time with him until Joe got up to make some salmon for dinner. Sitting in front of the television, they watched the news while they ate.

After dinner, they watched television and discussed the out-of-body episode. Joe said he wanted to get more regular with his meditation as it seemed to help clarify his thoughts as he did some. He felt that it would probably help to promote more OBEs over time. He excused himself and went to the easy chair in his study and tried some meditation for about half an hour. When he finished, he came back out to Mary, telling her that he felt he had a good meditation.

They felt it was time for bed, and Mary had calmed Sean down by letting him sit with them for a while. They put him to bed and climbed into bed themselves. They hugged each other and kissed before drifting off to sleep.

CHAPTER ELEVEN

A Working Weekend

The next morning arrived, and this was a Saturday that Mary worked, so she got ready for work along with Joe. A consultation for a patient with a bleeding disorder was called in to his service, and Dave saw the patient first. Once he had seen the patient, he presented him to Joe. Then all three of them, including John, went to see the patient, and labs were ordered. It could be a defect of clotting proteins or a platelet deficiency or dysfunction. Once they had finished their rounds, Joe and his crew said good-bye until tomorrow.

Joe got home and spent some time with Sean, who always loved the attention. He and Mary sat down to relax and chat. Joe mentioned his new consultation and what he thought it was going to turn out to be.

He then brought up the subject of his possible visitation by Anna and what it did to prevent him from getting really sick. He felt the episode was pretty close to being explained in no other way other than Anna showing up to warn him. However the process occurred, he wasn't sure about it, but it had to be a spirit-to-spirit interaction. How else could they communicate with each other?

Mary responded, "Are you sure that you didn't just react to your acute illness with a first symptom being a hallucination caused by the infection? Illnesses can be manifested in strange ways sometimes."

Joe answered, "It is possible that it was just that, but it seemed very real. And besides, it seems that the illness manifested as a communication from Anna before I had any other symptoms." He hoped that that was not going to be the only time that it was going to happen. Not only was it a nice experience, but it was informative as well.

Mary didn't have a problem with the visitation even though Joe had, in the past, loved Anna very much and was going to marry her at one time. There was no jealousy on Mary's part regarding Joe's past. In a way, it was nice for Joe to have the communication that he had with Anna.

Mary mentioned, "I took a trip to the grocery store for a few things, and we could eat something easy today, like a delivered pizza. Then tomorrow we could have a stew with the meat I bought today." That sounded good to Joe. He said that he could start the stew when he got back from the hospital.

They ordered the pizza a little later. Once they found a movie to watch on the television, they sat down to watch it while they enjoyed their pizza with Sean sitting between them, one of his favorite spots, second only to Mary's lap for comfort. Once the movie started, Sean seemed to become more relaxed, and he seemed ready for bed before long.

When the movie was over, it was time for some nightly news, so they watched that before going off to bed themselves. Mary and Joe hugged and held each other in bed until they felt ready to close their eyes. They kissed for a while and then drifted off to sleep for the night.

Once morning came, Joe arose from the bed to go to the hospital. When he was ready, he gave Mary a kiss good-bye and drove off to work. He picked up some coffee on the way for a boost with his rounds. The morning went well. The new patient with the clotting abnormality seemed to be improving, and Joe started him on some oral medicine in preparation for discharge in a couple of days. The rest of their patients seemed to be doing well, so once Joe was finished, he gave John a call to go over the patients on the phone. John had been in a little earlier, so he had seen the patients earlier.

Joe went home and had a little time to write some notes regarding the patients before getting started with preparing the stew meat for slow cooking to get it started for an early dinner. Once it was ready, with potatoes, carrots, and celery, they sat down to eat some dinner.

They finished dinner and discussed their day. Then they cleaned up and watched television for a while before putting Sean to bed for the night. They decided to go to bed early for some close time together. They removed each other's clothes and got under the covers together. Joe enjoyed removing Mary's clothes, finding it very stimulating.

They began with some hugs and kisses. Then Joe began to stroke Mary with a hand, which Mary seemed to find exciting and soothing at the same time. Mary returned the stroking with some passionate kissing, which Joe enjoyed. Mary began to coo with pleasure and got as close to Joe as she could. She began to feel a tingle throughout her as she responded to Joe's strokes.

She was returning the favor by rubbing Joe's chest and then his abdomen, which he was greatly enjoying.

Mary got on top of Joe, and he held her close as they became more intimate. Joe liked it when Mary would at times get on top and initiate the lovemaking. It made him tingle all over when she did that. He loved to have her weight on him while she pleasantly vocalized during their lovemaking. Once they were done, they kissed once more and then held each other until they were ready to roll on their backs and fall asleep.

The next morning, they rose together and prepared for work. They showered together so that they could kiss a little more before getting some clothes on for their day at the hospital. They dressed and had a bite to eat before Joe drove them to work. Once they arrived, they said their good-byes and went their separate ways.

Chapter Twelve

Another OBE Experience

A number of days passed without incident until Joe found himself having another out-of-body experience one afternoon while he had a short nap to get some energy to complete the day. When he was reawakened enough to go over the episode in his head, he began to piece the episode together. It was centered on a discussion with Anna again, wherein she helped him with a particularly difficult patient. She gave some insight into the patient's condition and the treatment needed for recovery. The answers appeared to make sense, so he followed Anna's recommendation.

He and Anna were able to relate how much they missed each other, but it was obvious to Anna in her ethereal state that he and Mary were happy with each other. Anna was able to relay her knowledge of Joe's present relationship with Mary, and she was happy for him. Anna also relayed her concern over Joe's health and told him to keep up with regular to doctor-patient interactions to keep a watch on his sarcoidosis.

The sarcoidosis had been under decent control without a need for draining abdominal fluid, and he was able to relieve his pain with pain medication. The pain lingered, however, and he needed something to lessen it. His cane made him feel safer when he was about, walking short distances. His longest distance was only about a block before he really felt tired out.

That time, during his out-of-body experience, he was able to go deeper, and he viewed the astral plane with a better understanding. He was able to travel to areas of space not normally available to a person otherwise living a normal life. It was not to say that these things didn't happen to most people. It was just that the experience was usually not remembered when one returned to the more normal waking state. Sometimes, though, the episode was remembered and retrieved when one woke up.

Because of the admonishment to watch his sarcoidosis, he made an appointment after talking to John about his concern over his illness. They scheduled it for the next day.

Later, when they were on their way home, Joe mentioned his decision and reasoning for seeing John the next day just for a checkup. Mary told Joe that it seemed like a good idea. When they got home, they spent some time with Sean. He seemed to be growing so quickly, now scooting more around the house. They then reheated the stew for an easy dinner, and then they sat with Sean for a while as they watched the news.

The evening was quiet, and Joe caught up on his journal reading while Mary got some laundry done. When it was time for bed, they disrobed and climbed into bed and fell asleep quickly after a few hugs and kisses.

Morning came, and they prepped for a trip to work after greeting Mary's mother, who came over as she did on workdays to watch Sean. They drove to work, and Mary went off to work while Joe went to the outpatient area where Joe had agreed to meet John.

Joe met John, and he started out reminding John why he had made an appointment. John looked at Joe, noting his liver to be a little bit enlarged as it had been before. All in all there were no new problems that John could find. He ordered some blood work, an EKG, and a chest x-ray to compare it to previous x-rays. Joe went down to the lab and x-ray to get those things done so that they could get results by the end of the day. They then went off together to make their rounds together.

The day at work was ending as Joe got a call from John about his lab results. His platelet count was a little low, probably related to his enlarged liver and possibly enlarged spleen. The chest x-ray Joe had taken a look at earlier showed a possible slightly worsening infiltrates and some abnormal mediastinal areas.

John suggested that because of his neuropathic pain, especially in his legs, and his worsening chest x-ray, they start a course of steroids to see if his symptoms and signs improve. Joe agreed, and John wrote a prescription for the steroids.

Joe related the results to Mary on their way home from work. After finding Sean, they sat down on the couch, and shortly after, they decided to order pizza for dinner, something simple.

After they read a little of Sean's favorite book to him, they put him to bed for the night. Mary put the leftover pizza in the refrigerator, and then they cozied up together while they watched a couple of their favorite television shows. After the nightly news, they went off to bed for a good night of sleep. They slept well, and when morning arrived, they were rested and ready to start their new day. Joe started his steroid medication, and he planned to check his blood sugar and electrolytes in a couple of weeks. They had decided on using the medication for two to three months, depending on how he felt and how he reacted to the medication. He hadn't had any trouble with it as he took it when he was first diagnosed with the sarcoidosis.

Once they were ready, they left for their day at work. Mary asked Joe, "How was your nighttime sleep?"

"It was calm," he replied. "No more traveling last night."

Mary answered, "I am not sure if that is a good thing or not."

Joe agreed, "Me too, but I think, over the long run, it is a good thing when I travel."

Mary and Joe went to the ninth floor, Mary to work the day there, Joe to find his residents so they could start rounding. They first saw those few patients that they needed hands on with so that they could then sit through the rest of the patients. They spent about an hour sitting while they went over those patients that they didn't see. When they finished, Joe asked if they missed anything or if there were any questions unanswered. Nothing came up, so rounds were over. Joe went to the library for an hour or so until Mary was done. She came to the library to pick up Joe, and they took off for home.

As always, they were happy to see and greet Sean. Mary played with him for a while and then sat with him as Joe put together a warm chicken salad. They moved to the couch, and Sean was fine with them while they ate the salad. After a little snack, Sean was ready for bed, so Joe took him off to bed and put him in pajamas. He rubbed him with a little, light pressure and said good night to Sean.

He went back to the couch to watch a little more television with Mary. They sat in each other's arms until after the news. Then they went off to bed to get some sleep.

CHAPTER THIRTEEN

A View of Time

"A few years ago, we had a discussion on the nature of time," Joe said. "But here, we are going to view time differently. It is not just linear or nonlinear. Time can become amorphous, a less controlled condition of time and space with some of its own rules."

It was about a week before their next debate, and Joe was talking to his residents as they stopped to catch lunch. Before they split up, Joe mentioned the time for the meeting and his decision to take the nature of time from a few years ago and discuss it in more depth. "As I mentioned, we discussed the nature of time and decided that it was nonlinear." The others liked the idea, and Joe decided to have John talk in favor of nonlinear, lobular time. "Tom here will argue in favor of linear time. Actually what is the character and stability of the shape of time?"

When they got together, it was decided to have John go first. He stood and began, "It was decided a few years ago that time was nonlinear rather than linear because of the need to assimilate or make sense of time. Linear time does not express the true nature of the existence of time. Because of the occasional glimpse of the future, linear time can't express the full nature of time. In order to do that, time has to be nonlinear, and all of time is available at once in order to access the greater existence that is all of time at once.

"This way we can view all of time at once, including the future. In order to do that, time must be a system of multiple times being played out at once. Then the movement through time is movement from one point in time to another point with the shift going from one moment to another without the linear nature being involved. I'll give the floor to Tom."

John sat, and Tom rose to speak. "Time here is by nature linear in the physical realm of existence. It appears to move from present to future in an intelligible way with the future occasionally butting in. Time needs to be linear for us to make sense of our physical existence. If time were nonlinear, we couldn't make sense of our existence. It would be a confused mess if tomorrow was experienced today and yesterday was experienced tomorrow or otherwise didn't happen yet. To us here now, time is moving from now to tomorrow, or we couldn't make any sense of today and tomorrow. Occasionally in a dream, time can seem to move nonlinearly, but that is an illusion in our dream state. We have to have time move linearly if we are going to grow older as each day appears to occur from day to day. I will give the floor back to John."

Tom sat down, and John stood and began, "Time occurs nonlinearly, but by convention, we arrange it to run linearly in the physical plane to make sense of it. On the mental plane, the same activities occur as on the physical plane, but it is not necessary to arrange the happenings linearly because that happens at the mental plane level where we assimilate what occurs on the physical plane and rearrange it to make sense of it in the physical plane. It flows linearly in the physical plane even if it isn't truly linear at the higher levels of awareness."

He gave the floor back to Tom, who rose again once John had sat back down. "John has given an explanation for nonlinear time that makes some sense, but it just seems more complicated than it needs to be. By just observing time, one has to accept linear time as the norm. We are born, grow old, and die. That is the nature of time, we need not experience a jumbled-up time that conforms to linear time only in our imagination. Linear time is real, and we accept it as it feels to be, linear. No special tricks in managing time are necessary. I will give the floor back to John if he has anything more to say."

As Tom sat, John rose again and asked the crowd, "Does anyone have questions or comments?"

Dave raised a hand, and when recognized, he asked, "You didn't reference the past. How does it fit into your scheme of nonlinear time?"

John answered, "The past is just like the present or the future. It is accessible and can be arranged into a linear memory. It is easier than the future because by convention, it has already occurred and can be more easily arranged. Singular memory of the past is easy because of the input of a singular past. A group past is more difficult because it can vary from person to person."

John continued, "I think that we are done with the discussion today, so I will officially end this for now." With that, the audience arose and filed out of the auditorium.

Joe caught John and Tom at the end and thanked them for an interesting discussion. He then caught up with Mary, and they left the hospital for the day. Mary told Joe that she had enjoyed the discussion.

They went home and greeted Sean, who smiled when he saw them. Joe prepared hamburgers for dinner. They sat down on their favorite couch and watched the news as they ate.

Joe told Mary that he thought that they should discuss his visitations at the next meeting. Mary thought that that would be interesting.

Once it got a little later, they put Sean to bed and returned to the couch for a while. As they watched television, they cuddled up together. After some late night television, they decided to go to bed for the night. Joe followed Mary into the bedroom, and they held each other and kissed for a while until they were ready to go to sleep for the night.

Chapter Fourteen

Another Visitation

A new day started, and after a couple of weeks, the steroids that Joe was taking seemed to lessen his neuropathic pain. When he mentioned this to John, John replied that they should take the steroids for about a month and start tapering it over the next couple of months. They could repeat the chest x-ray and the blood work then.

Joe agreed with the plan but said he would get a blood sugar done after the first month, just to be sure that he was okay with that. He hoped that he would get a lasting effect from the full course of steroids with a reduction in the pain and numbness in his legs.

Joe had a chance to tell Mary about his visit with John. Then he met up with his residents on the seventh floor. They did rounds together on their patients, and all were without any acute problems. Joe was feeling a little tired after yesterday's meeting in the auditorium, so he told Mary that he was going to go home early and come back for her when her shift ended.

When they got home, Joe went into the study and took a little nap before Mary made some fish with rice for dinner. Joe went to bed early to catch up on more sleep. During the night, he had another vivid dream involving Anna where she had discussed encephalopathy with him. He awakened with an upset stomach and no appetite. He then had an episode of hematemesis and realized that he was probably not feeling well because of some upper gastrointestinal bleeding and was beginning to feel encephalopathic. Instead of going in to work, they went to the emergency room, and from there, he was sent for an emergency endoscopy and given an intensive care bed for close observation. He had lost a couple of units of blood before they could get his bleeding stopped, so he was given some blood also to maintain his blood hemoglobin level.

He stabilized over the morning hours, but he was clearly having some encephalopathy, which was treated with an increase in his dose of lactulose, which helped the symptoms of confusion. He improved in general over the next few days, and he was more alert to his surroundings.

Again he credited Anna with giving him some warning about his bleeding complication. Her discussion of his encephalopathy was clearly predicted by Anna. He took it as another aid given to him to help catch his symptoms early.

Once he was doing better, he decided to ask Dave and Sandy if they would take the next debate. Once they heard that Joe wanted to discuss visitations from previously living people or people at the time of their death, Joe offered to discuss his experience with them when they wanted his input. They agreed to do the debate, and each wanted to hear Joe's experiences. Once it was nearing time for the discussion, Joe talked to them both about his experience with his grandfather's passing. At that time, he dreamed of his passing and then was called by his mother the next day to be informed of Grandpa's passing the night before.

His other experiences were better known because Joe had talked to several residents about the communications he was having from Anna, more or less regularly, about things in the present or things that occurred after her death. With this information, he had come to believe in the spirit or soul living beyond the physical existence. He believed in the ability to continue communicating with those who had already passed on.

When it was time for another debate, John asked Joe to give some remarks about his experiences. He related the remarks he had shared with Dave and Sandy and left the discussion with Dave to start the debate. Dave began by relating his understanding of Joe's comments. He sounded to be very sure of what he discussed, and it seemed to make sense to Dave. After Dave made a few comments, he concluded, "Joe should really have done this talk instead of me because we are essentially using his experiences to debate this side of the argument. I am going to give the floor to Sandy and say good luck, but I think Joe has my side of the argument sewn up."

Dave gave the floor to Sandy and sat down. Sandy stood, saying, "About the only way to argue this discussion is to say that Joe was hallucinating or dreaming when he had the experiences. Here is a place for wishful thinking. What more would Joe enjoy than more time with Anna, even if it is a hallucination or just a result of a strong desire to speak more with Anna. That is only natural."

Joe raised a hand, and when pointed to, he added, "The subjects were clear to me, and when related to my health, they were true with Anna. Her interventions helped with my care a few times. I am indebted to her."

The episodes with Anna were much more than a hallucination. They gave Joe a sense of being that was clear to him during his dream state. The incidents were occurring mostly when he fell off to sleep or when he awakened from a period of sleep.

He wasn't the only person this ever happened to. Anecdotes had been written often about episodes of out-of-body states, especially during sleep or while meditating.

As mentioned before, they could be in sleep states or during meditation. These states were reproducible, brought on at times by meditation or by the sleep state.

Some people, such as true mediums, have access to people who have passed on and can communicate with them bidirectionally. They can talk to each other. Specifically, the one still living learns a lot about the person they listen to, that they are in communication with. These communications are frequently full of information for the living listener.

So there are a lot of things said and learned from these communiqués. There's a lot learned when they communicate with each other.

A person learns from the person who has already passed.

Dave and Sunny had finished their talk, so they asked if there were other questions. A hand went up from one of the surgical residents. Dave pointed to him and asked, "Yes?"

The surgical resident asked, "What happens to the patient's psyche or soul when he is put to sleep during surgery?"

Dave answered, "There are several different possibilities mentioned. The patient could simply go to sleep. He could have cerebral hypoxia and be left with a feeling that he can't think right, or he could possibly have an out-of-body experience and have a memory of traveling great distances to varied locations."

Once questions were taken care of, John closed the meeting until next time, assuming nothing got in the way of their schedule.

The debate finished, Joe found Mary, and they grabbed something to eat for when they got home. They greeted Sean, and he was in his usual good mood. Mary fed him while Joe checked the mail, opening the important things. They then sat in front of the television while they worked on their sandwiches. Once it got later, Joe put Sean to bed and then came back to sit with Mary for a while longer.

Once the news was over, they went off to bed and crawled in together. They hugged and kissed for a while and then rolled over for some sleep.

CHAPTER FIFTEEN

Encephalopathy

They awakened the next day feeling pretty good. After their shower and something to eat, they got in the car for a ride to work. Joe encountered no surprises, which was how he liked it. Today was a day for teaching rounds with the residents, so he met them before lunch.

They rounded on the floor at first and then finished with the patients that Joe already knew last. There was a new patient on the floor with a fever of unknown origin. He had been pan-cultured and started on broad-spectrum antibiotics while the workup was continued. The patient grew more short of breath over the first day that he was in the hospital. The confusing part, initially, was that despite the appearance of the patient, he initially grew nothing on cultures until he grew pneumococci from his cerebrospinal fluid. Because of the unusual presentation with bacteria in his cerebrospinal fluid, he was worked up further. He had just six white blood cells in his spinal fluid, but that was a little abnormal as well. Over the next couple of days, a bone marrow biopsy showed abnormal white cells pointing toward a leukemic laden fluid, giving him a complication of an immunocompromised host, making him prone to infection due to the abnormal white blood cells.

So he was an immunocompromised host with leukemia underlying an infection in his cerebrospinal fluid, making him prone to infection. He was placed on more appropriate and specific antibiotics, and they all hoped and waited for improvement with the antibiotics if there was enough time to treat him before he succumbed to the infection. Over the next couple of days, it appeared that he was going to make it as he was responding well to the antibiotics.

The rest of the teaching rounds were unremarkable with no other surprises or diagnostic dilemmas. Once they finished teaching rounds, Joe was pretty much done with patient care for the day.

John had been busy with a consult for a high white blood cell count while the others had been having their teaching rounds. He met with Joe in the library to discuss the case. The patient was also being seen by the infectious disease service to help rule out infection as the source of the elevated white cell count. As before, the patient had been pan-cultured, and Joe decided they would do a bone marrow biopsy later that day. It appeared this time to be an infection, and the patient was placed on broad-spectrum antibiotics, waiting for cultures to grow something. Once the patient appeared to have sepsis, he was given to the infectious disease service for them to take care of him.

With the end of the discussion regarding the patient with sepsis, Joe's day was pretty much finished. He spent some time in the library again while he waited for Mary to finish her workday. When she saw him, he looked a little more tired than usual, which concerned her. They got in the car and stopped for a sandwich to have for dinner, and then they went home to Sean.

Sean had grown enough that he was starting to crawl around to go places in the house, so he needed closer attention to make sure that he didn't get into any trouble tooling around the house during the day. He was happy to sit with Joe for a while, so they buddied around while Mary got some clothes washed. Once they had put Sean to bed, they took their sandwiches to the couch and ate them in front of the television.

Joe was too tired to stay up for the nightly news, so he went to bed early. When morning came, Joe was feeling a little worse, so they called John to say that Joe wasn't going to work that day, but he wanted to see John as a patient. They agreed to meet at 10:00 AM so that John could check him out. On examination, Joe was showing some aggravation of his hepatic encephalopathy again, so he had cultures drawn once more.

John was concerned enough that he had Joe admitted and seen by the hepatologist that they knew and trusted. Joe was placed on treatment for worsening of his encephalopathy and had cultures taken to rule out infection. Antibiotics were started also to treat for infection and to help the encephalopathy.

It was becoming worrisome that he had an infection a couple of times recently. Consideration of removing his hepatojugular shunt was entertained, but they decided to try to treat the infection with intravenous antibiotics once more without removing and replacing the shunt as it seemed to be doing so well with managing his ascitic fluid.

Joe's encephalopathy manifested with confusion, first, about where he was and progressed to confusion about the time and date. Watching him over the next couple of days, though, showed some improvement with the antibiotics and increasing his medicine specifically for the encephalopathy. He grew gram-negative bacteria in his bladder, and he improved on the antibiotics. He figured he bit the bullet once more with his chronic illness. He was lucky once more.

After a few days, he had cleared enough to continue recovery at home. Mary drove him home, and over the next few days, she took over making meals and going to work on her own while Joe continued to recover at home.

As he got better, it was easy to tell once he began to argue that he was ready to get back to work. Although he went back too early for Mary, he did appear to function well enough to return to short days at work. He did feel more tired when he got home from work, but he felt that he was doing well enough to handle some short days, and he felt more productive once he was back at the hospital. There was only so much that he could do from home.

He continued to go to bed a little early, but Mary did follow him to bed a few nights when she could get Sean to bed early too. They were able to cuddle for a while in bed before going off to sleep.

Joe hoped that he would be able to continue working as a physician. He didn't plan on hanging up his stethoscope this early in his career. He wanted to follow his sarcoidosis and treat it for a while yet. He wasn't ready to quit yet, though he knew that John would take him on as a consultant in the office when he felt the need to slow down.

He made a note to himself to discuss the work options with John the next morning when they had some free time together. John reassured Joe that he would have a position in their medicine and hematology practice. He was reassured by the hospital administration that he could keep his practice until John was ready to join him in a practice together. They could then run their practice from the hospital. This was all reassuring to Joe as he felt that with this arrangement, he could provide for Mary and Sean and not tire himself out too much too soon.

Joe and Mary, finished with their workday, left the hospital, and went home to visit with Sean and have something to eat for dinner.

Chapter Sixteen

Another Bleeding Episode

Joe awakened the next morning. Mary had the day off, and Joe decided that he would take the day off as well so the three of them could take a playdate with Sean and enjoy a walk since it wasn't too cold for a wagon ride around the block. Sean was getting more alert to his surrounding environment, and he enjoyed the entertainment of watching a couple of squirrels cavorting around in the trees as well as from tree to tree. Joe felt that he was being watched by the squirrels, like he was being entertainment for them.

After they got back home, they put Sean back down to bed for a nap while they planned a night out for dinner and a movie. Since they had given Mary's mom the day off, they figured she would be okay with watching Sean so that they could go out on a date, which they hadn't done much since Sean came into their lives.

Joe took an afternoon nap to recharge his batteries for their evening out. He still was prone to tiring very easily without some extra afternoon naps.

He awakened around 4:00 PM and hopped into the shower to get cleaned up a bit for their night out. Mary showered after Joe and decided to wear the dress she bought to wear the night that they got engaged. Mary still had her stone, which she considered her first engagement stone from Joe, given to her before he offered her a real engagement ring.

Joe opened up the conversation by stating that he didn't think that he could continue on as a physician except for some severe restrictions on his work schedule. He said, "I think I could still do some consulting or clinic work. I'll just need to watch my fatigue level."

Mary replied, smirking, "As long as they let you hang around as a deadbeat physician who haunts the halls of the hospital, I guess they would let you hang around. If you give the medicine resident program a little aid if a resident drops by you for insight regarding aiding the residents, your actions would aid the patient as well."

Joe agreed and then concentrated on their dinner, planning to do better with their meal than on the night they got engaged. They finished up dinner and drove to the movie theater to catch a movie that Mary had been talking about seeing for a while.

With some popcorn and a drink of soda, they watched the movie. By the time it was over, they were anxious to get back home to Sean. They arrived home a little noisily, probably because Mary and Joe wanted to see Sean. He did awaken and called out to them to pick him up. Once the sleepiness cleared from his head, he greeted them with smiles and gurgles as he looked at them back home.

After a while in Mary's and Joe's laps, Sean was ready to return to bed for some more sleep. After Mary's mom camped out in their third bedroom for the night, Joe and Mary went off to bed as well.

A new morning arrived with some sunshine, and it looked like it was going to be a nice day. Joe decided to talk to John about limiting his workload as he had discussed with Mary. John seemed okay with the change and stated frankly, "I wondered when you were going to realize that you needed to take the work reduction in order to last a little longer."

Joe invited John over for hamburgers on the grill, and John accepted. Once John arrived for the evening, he and Joe talked about the changes they would have to make, which were really not much different. Joe was going to try to handle the new consultations and spend some time with the residents on an as-needed basis. He would be available when the residents had questions for their service, and that way, he could stay active in the residency program.

They had their meal, and John thanked Mary for the food. He asked Mary how she thought Joe was doing. She voiced some concerns and said she just wants to be sure that they keep Joe's work limited because he did tire out easily, and Sean was getting more active and needing more of their personal time with him. She wanted to impress John with Joe's responsibilities regarding Sean and wanted to be sure that Joe had the energy to help interact with Sean, especially while she was at work more than Joe was going to be. John was wholehearted when he responded that Sean should be Joe's priority while he was home.

They finished their dinner and discussion, mostly regarding Joe's condition, which made Joe uncomfortable. They said their good-byes, and John went off toward his home while Joe and Mary sat for a little bit, watching the tail end of the news. They then went off to bed once they were sure that Sean was sleeping comfortably. After some hugs and kisses, they closed their eyes for the night.

In the middle of the night, Joe awakened with some nausea, which progressed to some coffee-ground-appearing emesis. He was also acting a little more confused than when they had gone off to sleep. Mary didn't bother to ask Joe but, instead, just called her mom to come over because they needed her to watch Sean while they went off to the emergency room to evaluate and treat Joe's acute upper gastrointestinal bleeding. Once Mary's mom arrived, Mary drove Joe to the hospital for an evaluation of his bleeding. Once the hospital staff saw him arrive, they called for an intensive care bed.

They consulted Joe's GI service as well to fill them in on Joe's present state. Joe was prepped for an upper endoscopy first thing in the morning after he was stabilized with a blood transfusion. The upper scope showed that one of his esophageal varices, which had been previously banded, was starting to leak some blood. The lesion was banded once more as the amount of bleeding at the time was minimal. Joe seemed to tolerate the procedure well, but he began having significantly more encephalopathy because of the blood in his gastrointestinal tract. He was treated aggressively, and the bleeding appeared to have stopped after the variceal banding.

The doctor, GI doctor, did the procedure and then came out to find Mary to talk to her. He impressed on her that any bleeding episodes could be life threatening, and even though his episode seemed to have responded to the endoscopy, any one of an episode could be life threatening, and he should think through his work decision deeply.

Mary agreed to discuss work with Joe when he was feeling better. She promised also to do her best about getting Joe to take some vacation time. She felt that some special time with Sean would help to calm Joe down for a while. To Mary's surprise, it wasn't difficult to talk Joe into taking the time. She told him he could write some of his thoughts about Sean down. This was something that he had wanted to start—to have something for Sean about his early childhood when he got older.

Joe had long felt that Sean was somehow aware of himself more than the average child of his age. Joe had felt a significant relationship between the three of them, thinking that they might have had a relationship before their present births and the interactions that they had with each other.

He could relate to this interaction as if they all three had agreed to try this present time that they were having together. As the days at home continued on, Joe felt that he was gaining more insights as to how Sean interacted with them. Joe didn't think he was just being a doting parent but felt that Sean was communicating nonverbally often—more than one would expect for someone just months old.

This communication seemed precocious from Joe's viewpoint, but he felt it was real. Joe had lightly dreamed of talking to Sean in an afternoon nap. During that time, Joe was given some insights into Sean's and Joe's future from Sean's viewpoint. Joe felt that in order to protect him, he was shown just part of his future, leaving some questions about his future untold. He liked what he saw in Sean's future except for an early loss of his father figure. Joe wasn't sure that he wouldn't leave this world in the near future, leaving Mary and Sean alone.

Joe greatly appreciated that he had these days with Sean, watching him grow and change. He suddenly developed some nausea and blood per rectum. He called Mary and told her. She dashed home and took him to the emergency room for evaluation and admission once again. He was also showing encephalopathic symptoms, so it was good that Mary was with him. He was evaluated and sent for an emergency upper endoscopy and placed into the intensive care unit for observation.

Mary tried to tell Sean about his father's condition, and Sean acted as if he understood, not wanting to know his condition, turning away from Mary when she talked to him. Again it seemed to Mary that Sean shouldn't understand what she was saying, but he appeared to be acting appropriately for the situation, though he should be too young to understand.

Joe's hospital stay was more prolonged this time, with a repeat endoscopy before he was discharged from intensive care to spend some time monitoring his counts on the medical floor.

Epilogue

A Conversation

With many of his encephalopathic dreams during the day and the dreams at night, Joe met with Sean, who told him that where they were was an interim area sometimes still reachable by a young child or a severely ill person or soul from the souls' grouping. He was being contacted by the helper soul, and he was doing his best to help find the way through this path, which was generally lost after the onset of older childhood was entered. The ability was lost to contact this area, which had soul-group souls planning their next incarnation. It was the time between lives. It manifested at the beginning and ending of the life, and for those near the edges of their life, it was also more commonly experienced.

Here, decisions were made on what the things in the earthly existence of physical life were going to be like, what was going to be learned. This was all for learning what lessons we were capable of dealing with during each life. The life's plan was then created.

Sean continued, "I am lucky to have kept my soul awareness as long and as active as I have. It gives me a wider view of time, and here I know a few extra things about time and how the lives fit together. We are undergoing a large learning experience while we are here in our earthly existences.

"Dad, I will see you again, and you will see me again. That much I know."